The Ultimate Guide to Vegetarian Meals

Amazing Vegetarian Recipes for the Whole Day

America Best Recipes

Table of Contents

Breakfast
No-bake keto granola bars with peanut butter

No-bake keto granola bars peanut butter, easy healthy granola bars. Creamy peanut butter, flaxseed meal, chia seeds, almonds, coconut and more! 100% Sugar free, gluten free paleo breakfast or snacks.

Prep Time: 10 mins Total Time: 30 mins

Servings: 8 breakfast bars

Ingredients

Wet ingredients

1/2 cup Natural Peanut butter or almond butter if paleo
1/4 cup Coconut oil

2 teaspoons Vanilla extract

Dry ingredients

1/3 cup Erythritol - like erythritol

1/2 cup Sliced almonds + extra 1 tablespoon to decorate on top 1/3 cup Flaxseed meal

1 tablespoon Chia seeds 1/3 cup Pumpkin seeds

1/4 cup Unsweetened desiccated Coconut 1/2 teaspoon Cinnamon

Chocolate drizzle

3 tablespoons Sugar-free Chocolate Chips

1 teaspoon Coconut oil

Instructions

Line a loaf pan, size 9 inches x 5 inches, with parchment paper. Set aside.

In a medium mixing bowl or a saucepan, place all the wet ingredients: peanut butter, coconut oil, and vanilla.

Microwave by 30 seconds burst, stir and repeat until the coconut oil is fully melted and combines with the nut butter. It should not take more than 1 minute 30 seconds. Otherwise, melt the ingredients in a saucepan under medium heat, stirring often to prevent the mixture from sticking to the pan.

Stir in the sugar-free crystal sweetener, stir and microwave an extra 30 seconds to incorporate well.

Erythritol doesn't dissolve very well but it will give some delicious sweet crunch into your bars or see paleo note.

In a large mixing bowl, add the rest of the dry ingredients: sliced almonds, flaxseed meal, chia seeds, pumpkin seeds, shredded coconut, and cinnamon. Stir to combine.

Pour the nut butter mixture onto the dry ingredients. Stir with a spatula to combine. You want to cover all the dry ingredients with the nut butter mixture.

Transfer the mixture into the prepared loaf pan. Press evenly the mixture with your hand to leave no air. Flatten the surface with a spatula.

Freeze for 20 minutes until the breakfast bars are hard and set. Remove from the freezer, lift the parchment paper to pull out the bar from the loaf pan. Place on a plate. Sprinkle extra sliced almonds on top.

In a small bowl, microwave the sugar-free dark chocolate and coconut oil until fully melted.

Drizzle the melted chocolate on top of the bar, return into the freezer 1-3 minutes until the chocolate is set.

Cut into 8 breakfast bars.

Wrap each bar individually into plastic wrap or bee wax. Store in the fridge up to 8 days.

Nutrition Info

Calories 306 Calories from Fat 253 Fat 28.1g Carbohydrates 9.6g Fiber 6.8g Sugar 1.4g Protein 7.9g

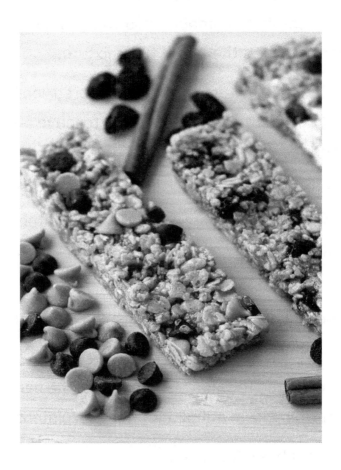

Cauliflower Tortillas

Prep Time 20minutes Cook Time 20 minutes Total Time 40minutes

Ingredients

Cauliflower Tortillas / Wraps

1 1/2 lb Cauliflower (florets only - about one large head)
3 large Egg

3/4 cup Mozzarella cheese (shredded) 1/2 tsp Sea salt

1/2 tsp Xanthan gum Spicy Low Carb Quesadilla Sauce

6 tbsp Mayonnaise

2 tbsp Jalapenos in water (from a jar, minced, with liquid included - equivalent to 2-3 slices + liquid)

3/4 tsp Paprika

1/2 tspGarlic powder Cayenne pepper (to taste)

Cheese Filling

1 1/2 cup Cheddar cheese (shredded)

Instructions

Preheat the oven to 400 degrees F (204 degrees C). Line two baking sheets with parchment paper.

Pulse the cauliflower florets in a food processor until they are the consistency of rice. (Use the grate attachment if you have one.)

Transfer to a large bowl and microwave on high for 8-10 minutes (or steam using your favorite method), until cooked.

Cool until the cauliflower is cool enough to handle. Transfer to a cheese cloth or towel and squeeze tightly to get rid of as much extra liquid as possible. It should be dense and clumpy.

Switch the food processor to the S blade and place the cauliflower back in. Add the eggs, mozzarella and salt. Process until smooth.

Sprinkle the xanthan gum on top (do not dump it in one clump). Process until smooth.

Drop the cauliflower mixture into six areas on the lined baking sheets. Use a spatula or the back of a spoon to spread into thin circles. Bake for 8-10 minutes, until the edges are dry and the bottom is golden. (If both baking sheets don't fit in the oven side by side, do one at a time.)

Carefully flip over, then bake for 4-6 more minutes. Cool for 10 minutes before moving.

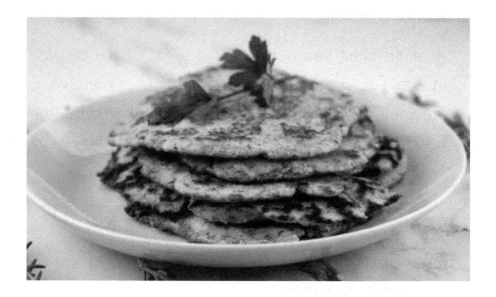

Low Carb Quesadillas

To make the sauce, whisk all ingredients in a small container. Cover and refrigerate to allow the flavors to develop (you can do this overnight if you have time).

Spread a tablespoon of the sauce over each cauliflower tortilla. Sprinkle 1/4 cup of shredded cheddar cheese on top. Fold in half.

Heat an oiled pan over medium heat. Place two folded quesadillas in the pan. Fry for a couple of minutes, until browned, then flip and repeat on the other side. Repeat with the remaining quesadillas.

Nutrition Info

Calories 108 Fat 5g Protein 9g Total Carbs 7g Net Carbs 4g Fiber 3g Sugar 3g

Detox Cauliflower Mushroom Bowls Recipe

Prep Time: 15 m Cook Time: 30 m 4 Servings

Ingredients

For the pesto:

1/4 cup Almonds, About 42 grams

1 cup Fresh Cilantro, Packed and roughly chopped, plus additional for garnish

For the bowl:

1/4 cup Fresh Mint, Lightly packed and roughly chopped
1/2 tablespoon Minced Fresh Jalapeño

1 teaspoon Fresh Lime Juice 1/4 teaspoon Salt

pinch of Black Pepper

1 tablespoon Extra Virgin Olive Oil

6 cups Cauliflower Florets

2 tablespoons Extra Virgin Olive Oil, Divided Salt and Pepper

3 cups Cremini Mushrooms

2 teaspoons Minced Fresh Garlic 8 cups Spinach, Packed

1/2 cup Pomegranate Seeds

Instructions

Pre heat your oven to 375°F. Spread the almonds onto a small baking sheet and bake until golden brown and "nutty" smelling, about 7-10 minutes. Set aside.

Place the cauliflower into a large food processor and process until rice-like.

Heat 1 tablespoon of the olive oil in a large pan over medium heat and add in the cauliflower rice and a pinch of salt and pepper. Cover and cook, stirring occasionally until lightly golden brown, about 10 minutes.

Heat 1 tablespoon olive oil in a separate medium pan on medium heat. Add in the sliced mushrooms, garlic, and a pinch of salt and pepper, and cook, stirring occasionally, until the mushrooms are golden brown and fork tender, about 8-10 minutes.

While the vegetables cook, add the toasted almonds into a SMALL food processor (mine is 3 cups) and pulse until broken down into small crumbs. Add in the cilantro, mint, jalapeno, lime juice, salt, and pepper and process until the herbs are broken down.

With the food processor running, stream in 2 tablespoons water and olive oil, stopping to scrape down the sides as necessary, until the pesto is smooth and creamy.

Add the spinach into the pot with the cauliflower rice (but don't mix it in, just let it sit on top of the cauliflower) and cover. Let the spinach sit for 2-3 minutes until it lightly wilts.

Divide the spinach between 4 bowls, followed by the cauliflower rice, mushrooms, and the pesto. Finally, sprinkle the pomegranate seeds on top and garnish with extra cilantro.

Mix around and DEVOUR!

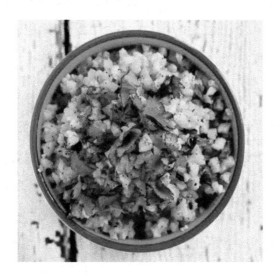

Zucchini & Sweet Potato Latkes

Servings: (4) 5" latkes

Ingredients

1 cup shredded zucchini

1 cup shredded sweet potato 1 egg, beaten

1 Tbsp coconut flour 1/2 tsp garlic powder 1/4 tsp ground cumin 1/2 tsp dried parsley Salt & pepper to taste

1 Tbsp ghee or clarified butter 1 Tbsp EV olive oil

Instructions

Combine the zucchini, sweet potato and egg in a medium bowl. In a small bowl, mix the coconut flour and spices together. Add the dry ingredients to the zucchini mixture and stir until fully combined.

Heat the ghee and olive oil in a medium nonstick pan. Divide the mixture into four equal portions and drop into the pan, pressing down with a fork until a 1/2 inch thick cake is formed. Cook on medium heat until golden and crisp, then flip carefully and cook the other side. Remove to a plate lined with paper towels to drain.

Season with an additional sprinkle of kosher salt. Serve hot.

Nutrition Info

Serving Size: 1 latke Calories: 122 Fat: 9g Carbohydrates: 6.25g net Protein: 3g

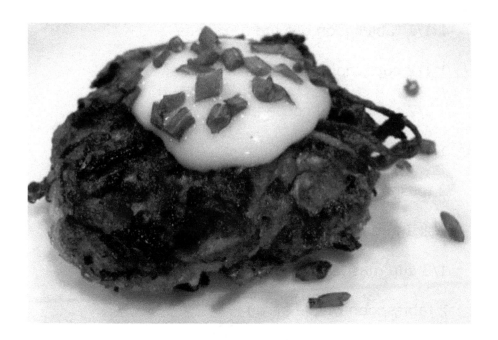

Chocolate Chip, Strawberry and Oat Waffles

Preparation time: 10 minutes Cooking time: 25 minutes Servings: 6

Ingredients:

6 tablespoons chocolate chips, semi-sweet

½ cup chopped strawberries

Powdered sugar as needed for topping

Dry 1/4 cup oats

1 1/2 tablespoon ground flaxseeds

1 1/2 cup whole wheat pastry flour

2 1/2 tablespoon cocoa powder

1/4 teaspoon salt

2 teaspoons baking powder

Wet Ingredients:

1/3 cup mashed bananas

2 tablespoon maple syrup

2 tablespoon coconut oil

1/2 teaspoon vanilla extract, unsweetened

1/4 cup applesauce, unsweetened

1 3/4 cup almond milk, unsweetened

Directions:

Take a medium bowl, place all the dry ingredients in it, and whisk until mixed. Take a large bowl, place all the wet ingredients in it, whisk until combined, and then whisk in dry ingredients mixture in four batches until incorporated, don't overmix.

Let the batter stand at room temperature for 5 minutes and in the meantime, switch on the waffle iron and let it preheat until hot. Then ladle one-sixth of the batter in it and cook until golden brown and firm.

Cook remaining waffles in the same manner and when done, top them with chocolate chips and berries, sprinkle with sugar and then serve

Sweet Potato and Apple Latkes

Preparation time: 5 minutes Cooking time: 15 minutes Servings: 4

Ingredients:

1 large sweet potato, peeled, grated

1/2 of medium white onion, diced

1 apple, peeled, cored, grated

2 tablespoons spelt flour

1 tablespoon arrowroot powder

½ teaspoon cracked black pepper

1 teaspoon salt

1 teaspoon turmeric

1 tablespoon olive oil and more for frying Tahini lemon drizzle, for serving

Directions:

Wrap grated potato and apple in a cheesecloth, squeeze moisture as much as possible, and then place it in a bowl. Add remaining ingredients and then stir until combined.

Take a skillet pan, place it over medium-high heat, add oil and when hot, drop in prepared batter, shape them into a round patty and cook for 4 minutes per side until crispy and brown. Serve latkes with Tahini lemon drizzle.

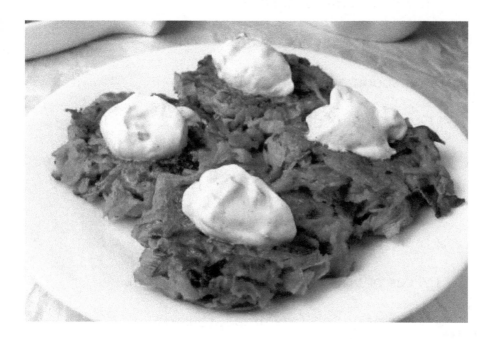

Vegan Breakfast Sandwich

Preparation time: 15 minutes Cooking time: 8 minutes

Servings: 3

Ingredients:

1 cup of spinach

6 slices of pickle 14 oz tofu, extra-firm, pressed

2 medium tomatoes, sliced

1/2 teaspoon garlic powder

¼ teaspoon ground black pepper

1/2 teaspoon black salt

1 teaspoon turmeric

1 tablespoon coconut oil

2 tablespoons vegan mayo

3 slices of vegan cheese

6 slices of gluten-free bread, toasted

Directions:

Cut tofu into six slices, and then season its one side with garlic, black pepper, salt, and turmeric.

Take a skillet pan, place it over medium heat, add oil and when hot, add seasoned tofu slices in it, season side down, and cook for 3 minutes until crispy and light brown.

Then flip the tofu slices and continue cooking for 3 minutes until browned and crispy. When done, transfer tofu slices on a baking sheet, in the form of a set of two slices side by side, then top each set with a cheese slice and broil for 3 minutes until cheese has melted.

Spread mayonnaise on both sides of slices, top with two slices of tofu, cheese on the side, top with spinach, tomatoes, pickles, and then close the sandwich. Cut the sandwich into half and then serve.

Tofu Scramble

Preparation time: 5 minutes Cooking time: 18 minutes Servings: 4

Ingredients:

For The Spice Mix:

1 teaspoon black salt

1/4 teaspoon garlic powder

1 teaspoon red chili powder

1 teaspoon ground cumin

3/4 teaspoons turmeric

2 tablespoons nutritional yeast

For The Tofu Scramble:

2 cups cooked black beans

16 ounces tofu, firm, pressed, drained

1 chopped red pepper

1 1/2 cups sliced button mushrooms

1/2 of white onion, chopped

1 teaspoon minced garlic

1 tablespoon olive oil

Directions:

Take a skillet pan, place it over medium-high heat, add oil and when hot, add onion, pepper, mushrooms, and garlic and cook for 8 minutes until golden. Meanwhile, prepare the spice mix and for this, place all its ingredients in a bowl and stir until combined. When vegetables have cooked, add tofu in it, crumble it, add black beans, sprinkle with prepared spice mix, stir and cook for 8 minutes until hot. Serve straight away

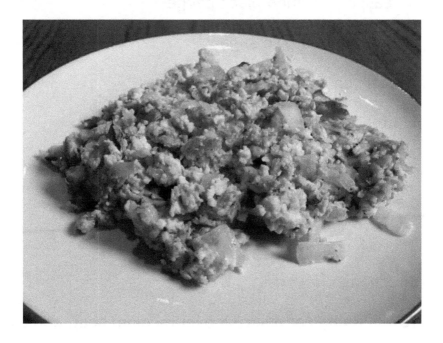

Chickpeas On Toast

Preparation time: 5 minutes Cooking time: 15 minutes
Servings: 6

Ingredients:

14-oz cooked chickpeas

1 cup baby spinach

1/2 cup chopped white onion

1 cup crushed tomatoes

½ teaspoon minced garlic

¼ teaspoon ground black pepper

1/2 teaspoon brown sugar

1 teaspoon smoked paprika powder

1/3 teaspoon sea salt

1 tablespoon olive oil

6 slices of gluten-free bread, toasted

Directions:

Take a frying pan, place it over medium heat, add oil and
when hot, add onion and cook for 2 minutes. Then stir in

garlic, cook for 30 seconds until fragrant, stir in paprika and continue cooking for 10 seconds. Add tomatoes, stir, bring the mixture to simmer, season with black pepper, sugar, and salt and then stir in chickpeas. Sir, in spinach, cook for 2 minutes until leaves have wilted, then remove the pan from heat and taste to adjust seasoning. Serve cooked chickpeas on toasted bread

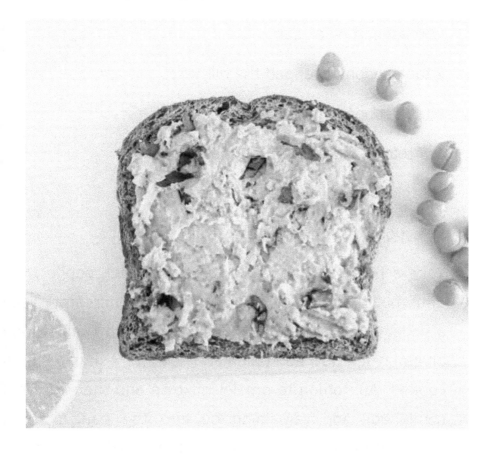

Chickpea Omelet

Preparation time: 5 minutes Cooking time: 10 minutes

Servings: 1

Ingredients:

3 Tablespoon chickpea flour

1 small white onion, peeled, diced

½ teaspoon black salt

2 tablespoons chopped the dill

2 tablespoons chopped basil

1/8 teaspoon ground black pepper

2 Tablespoon olive oil 8 Tablespoon water

Directions:

Take a bowl, add flour in it, salt and black pepper, stir until mixed, and then whisk in water until creamy. Take a skillet pan, place it over medium heat, add 1 tablespoon oil and when hot, add onion and cook for 4 minutes until cooked. Add onion to omelet mixture and then stir until combined. Add remaining oil into the pan, pour in prepared batter, spread evenly, and cook for 3 minutes per side until cooked. Serve omelet with bread.

Lunch
Mushroom Risotto
Prep time: 5 min Cooking Time: 30 min serve: 2

Ingredients

1 1/2 tablespoons avocado oil

1 cup mushrooms, sliced

1 tablespoon soy sauce

1 medium onion, finely diced

½ cup Arborio rice

½ teaspoon cumin seed

2 cups vegetable broth

½ cup grated parmesan

Salt and pepper to taste

¼ cup chopped cilantro

Instructions

Add ½ tablespoon avocado oil to the Instant Pot. Using the display panel select the Sauté function and adjust to More or High.

When oil gets hot, add sliced mushrooms. Cook, occasionally stirring for 7 minutes, then drain off any excess liquid.

Add soy sauce and cook and stir for an additional 7 minutes.

Add 1 tablespoon avocado oil to the Instant Pot and add rice and cumin seed to the Instant Pot and cook and stir 3 minutes.

Add vegetable broth and stir. Turn the pot off by selecting Cancel, secure the lid, and make sure the vent is closed.

Using the display panel, select the Manual or Pressure Cook function. Use the + /- keys and program the Instant Pot for 6 minutes.

When the time is up, quickly release the remaining pressure.

Stir risotto until desired consistency is reached about 2-3 minutes, returning to Sauté mode as needed.

Stir in parmesan cheese until melted. Adjust seasonings as needed.

Serve immediately garnished with chopped cilantro.

Nutrition Facts

Calories 278, Total Fat 4.3g, Saturated Fat 1.6g, Cholesterol 5mg, Sodium 1289mg, Total Carbohydrate 46.6g, Dietary Fiber 3.3g, Total Sugars 3.8g, Protein 12.7g

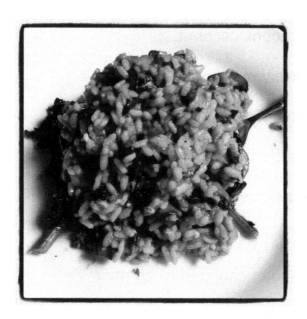

Buckwheat Tabbouleh

Prep time: 10 min Cooking Time: 15 min serve: 2

Ingredients

1 cup water

½ cup buckwheat

1 pinch salt

2 tablespoons coconut oil

½ tablespoon lemon juice

1 tomato, diced

½ cucumber, diced

¼ cup green onions, diced

1 carrot, grated

1 tablespoon chopped fresh mint

Instructions

Add buckwheat and water to the Instant Pot, secure the lid, and make sure the vent is closed.

Using the display panel, select the Manual or Pressure Cook function. Use the + /- keys and program the Instant Pot for 4 minutes.

When the time is up, let the pressure naturally release for 10 minutes, quickly releasing the remaining pressure.

Meanwhile, in a large bowl, combine coconut oil, sea salt, lemon juice, tomatoes, cucumber, green onions, carrots, and mint. Stir in cooled buckwheat.

Nutrition Facts

Calories 330, Total Fat 15.3g, Saturated Fat 12.2g, Cholesterol 0mg, Sodium 114mg, Total Carbohydrate 40.4g, Dietary Fiber 7g, Total Sugars 5.1g, Protein 7.5g

Carrot Rice

Prep time: 15 min Cooking Time: 15 min serve: 2

Ingredients

½ cup basmati rice

1 cup water

1/8 cup roasted peanuts

1 small onion, sliced

¼ teaspoon ginger powder

½ cup grated carrot

Salt to taste

Black pepper to taste

Chopped fresh parsley

Instructions

Grind peanuts in a blender and set aside. Select Sauté and add the onion; cook and stir until the onion has softened and turned golden brown about 10 minutes.

Stir in ginger powder, carrots, and salt to taste. Stir in black pepper and peanuts. Add rice and water combine.

Cover with the lid and make sure the vent is set to —Sealing‖. Pressure Cook on High for 5 minutes. Allow the steam pressure to release naturally for 5 minutes, then release any remaining pressure manually.

Garnish with chopped cilantro.

Nutrition Facts

Calories 249, Total Fat 4.9g, Saturated Fat 0.7g, Cholesterol 0mg, Sodium 108mg, Total Carbohydrate 44.9g, Dietary Fiber 3g, Total Sugars 3.3g, Protein 6.5g

Spinach Falafel

These green Spinach Falafel are vegan and gluten-free. Canned chickpeas are used for the base. They're baked in the oven with minimal oil. So good!

Prep Time 5 mins Cook Time 30 mins Total Time 35 mins Servings 12 falafel

Ingredients

17 oz canned chickpeas – rinsed and drained 2 cups fresh spinach

2 tablespoons besan/chickpea flour 3/4 teaspoon salt

baking spray

Instructions

Preheat the oven to 350°F/180°C.

Add the canned chickpeas, spinach, chickpea flour and salt to a food processor and blitz until combined. The mixture should stick together enough to form patties, if it doesn't add more chickpea flour.

Use an ice cream scoop to scoop the falafel on a baking tray lined with parchment paper. Press them a bit flatter and spray them with oil.

Bake them in the oven for about 30 minutes, carefully flipping them with a spatula after 20 minutes. They should be crispy on the outside and soft but not mushy on the inside.

Nutrition Info

Calories: 41kcal Carbohydrates: 6g Protein: 2g Sodium: 261mg Potassium: 96mg Fiber: 2g Calcium: 19mg Iron: 0.7mg

Roasted Turnips and Butternut Squash

Ingredients

3   medium tomatoes, cut into 1-inch pieces

1/2 butternut squash - peeled, seeded, and cut into 1-inch pieces

1 red onion, diced

1 turnip, peeled, and cut into 1-inch cubes

2 large carrots, cut into 1 inch pieces

2 large kohlrabi, cut into 1 inch pieces

3 tablespoons extra virgin olive oil

Seasoning ingredients

1 teaspoon salt

1/2 teaspoon ground black pepper

1 teaspoon onion powder

2 teaspoon garlic powder

1 teaspoon dried thyme

Garnishing Ingredients

2 sprigs fresh thyme, chopped (optional)

Directions:

Preheat your oven to 350 degrees F. Grease your baking pan. Combine the main ingredients on the prepared sheet pan. Drizzle with the oil and toss to coat. Combine the seasoning ingredients in a bowl. Sprinkle them over the vegetables on the pan and toss to coat with seasonings. Bake in the oven for 25 minutes. Stir frequently until vegetables are soft and lightly browned and chickpeas are crisp, for about 20 to 25 minutes more. Season with more salt and black pepper to taste, top with the thyme before serving.

Roasted Brussel Sprouts and Choy Sum

Ingredients

1 tablespoon extra virgin olive oil

8 cloves garlic, minced

1/2 teaspoon sea salt

1/4 teaspoon rainbow peppercorns

3 1/2 cups sliced choy sum

2 1/2 cups sliced Brussels sprouts

1 lime, cut into wedges

1 tablespoon chopped fresh cilantro

Directions:

Preheat your oven to 450 degrees F. Line a baking sheet with foil and grease with olive oil. Mix the olive oil, garlic, salt, and pepper in a bowl. Add in the choy sum and Brussel sprouts. Combine until well coated. Spread them out in a single layer on the baking sheet. Add the lime wedges. Roast in the oven until vegetables become caramelized for about 25 minutes. Take out the lime wedges and top with the cilantro.

Greek Quinoa

Prep time: 15 min Cooking Time: 10 min serve: 2

Ingredients

1 cup quinoa

1 tablespoon butter

2 cups vegetable broth

¼ teaspoon Greek seasoning

¼ teaspoon dried oregano

1/8 teaspoon salt

¼ cup pitted olives, drained and chopped

¼ cup chopped red peppers

¼ cup green peas

Crumbled goat cheese (optional)

Chopped fresh Italian parsley

Instructions

Rinse quinoa well; drain in a fine-mesh strainer.

Press Sauté; melt butter in Instant Pot. Add quinoa; cook 5 to 6 minutes or until golden brown, stirring occasionally. Add broth, green peas, red peppers,

Greek seasoning, oregano, and salt; mix well.

Secure lid and move pressure release valve to Sealing. Press Manual or Pressure Cook; cook at High Pressure 4 minutes.

When cooking is complete, use natural release for 10 minutes, then release

remaining pressure.

Stir in olives; garnish with cheese and parsley.

Nutrition Facts

Calories 511, Total Fat 19.3g, Saturated Fat 8.4g, Cholesterol 30mg, Sodium 1177mg, Total Carbohydrate 61.7g, Dietary Fiber 7.9g, Total Sugars 3.1g, Protein 22.9g

Minty Pea Risotto

Prep time: 10 min Cooking Time: 20 min serve: 2

Ingredients

2 tablespoons coconut oil

1 medium onion, peeled and diced

½ teaspoon garlic powder

½ cup barley

1 cup vegetable broth, divided

¼ teaspoon salt

1/8 teaspoon ground black pepper

¼ teaspoon lime zest

¼ cup chopped fresh mint leaves

½ cup fresh peas

1 carrot

Instructions

Press the Sauté button to the Instant Pot. Add coconut oil to the Instant Pot and heat 30 seconds. Add onion and stir-fry for 5 minutes until they are translucent. Add garlic powder and barley and cook for an additional minute. Add ½ cup broth and stir for 3 minutes until it is absorbed by barley. Add remaining cup broth, salt, and pepper. Lock lid. Press the Manual or Pressure Cook button and adjust the cooking time to 10 minutes. When the timer beeps, let the pressure release naturally for 10 minutes. Quickly release any additional pressure until the float valve drops and then unlock the lid.

Stir in lime zest, mint, carrot, and peas. Heat them for 3 minutes until peas are heated through.

Serve warm.

Nutrition Facts

Calories 372, Total Fat 15g, Saturated Fat 12g, Cholesterol 0mg, Sodium 590mg, Total Carbohydrate

50.3g, Dietary Fiber 13.2g, Total Sugars 7.4g, Protein 9.1g

Jackfruit Biryani

Prep time: 25 min Cooking Time: 30 min serve: 2

Ingredients

2 cups jackfruit cubes

1 cup basmati rice

½ cup coconut oil

¼ cup coconut milk

1 medium onion, thinly sliced

1 medium tomato, chopped

½ teaspoon ginger powder

½ teaspoon garlic powder

¼ cup plain yogurt beaten

¼ cup mint, chopped

1/8 cup walnut

1/8 cup raisins

¼ cup fried onions

Spice mix

1 teaspoon cumin seed

1 teaspoon coriander powder

½ teaspoon turmeric powder

½ teaspoon ginger powder

¼ teaspoon cinnamon powder

1/8 teaspoon black pepper, freshly ground

1/8 teaspoon nutmeg, freshly ground

¼ teaspoon cardamom, ground

Instructions

Wash and soak the rice in cold water.

Turn the Instant Pot to —Sauté‖ and add 1/2 tablespoon coconut oil. When

—Hot‖ and the chopped onions and sauté until light brown, about 3 minutes.

Add the jackfruit, ginger powder and garlic powder, and spice mix. Stir everything together, making sure the spice mix is evenly mixed with everything else. Sauté for 5 minutes.

Add 1/2 cup of water and mix well. Put on Pressure Cook for 10 minutes. This step makes the jackfruit nice and tender. Release pressure and open the lid carefully.

Add the yogurt, tomatoes, walnuts, and raisins. Mix everything. Add the soaked rice on top of the jackfruit mixture, spread it to make a thin layer of rice. Add 1/2 cup water and 1/2 cup coconut milk or 1 cup water. The water should just cover the rice layer. Put on pressure cook for 10 minutes.

Let pressure release naturally. Once released, carefully open the lid. Mix everything.

Serve in a bowl, garnish with fried onions and coriander.

Nutrition Facts

Calories 776, Total Fat 20.6g, Saturated Fat 13.8g, Cholesterol 2mg, Sodium 43mg, Total Carbohydrate

132.8g, Dietary Fiber 8g, Total Sugars 11.8g, Protein 14.9g

Lemon Tofu "Fried Rice" Casserole

Prep time: 10 min Cooking Time: 15 min serve: 2

Ingredients

1 tablespoon coconut oil

2 medium onion, trimmed and thinly sliced

½ teaspoon ginger, minced

1 teaspoon lemon zest, finely minced

2 cups Tofu

½ cup raw long-grain brown rice

1 cup vegetable broth

1/8 cup soy sauce

1/8 cup fresh lemon juice

½ tablespoon apple cider vinegar

½ teaspoon honey

Instructions

Press Sauté, set the time for 35 minutes. Warm the coconut oil in an Instant Pot for a minute or two. Add the onion, ginger, and zest of lemon. Cook, often stirring, just until the onions begin to soften about 1 minute. Add the tofu and cook, occasionally stirring until brown about 2 minutes. Add the rice and stir well until the grains are uniformly distributed throughout. Pour in the broth, turn off the Sauté function, and scrape up every speck of browned stuff on the pot's bottom. Stir in the soy sauce, lemon juice, honey, and vinegar until uniform. Lock the lid onto the cooker. Press Pressure Cook on Max Pressure for 10 minutes with the Keep Warm setting off. Use the Quick Release method to bring the Instant Pot's pressure back to normal, but do not open the cooker. Set it aside with the lid latched and the pressure valve open for 10 minutes. Unlatch the lid, open the pot, and stir well before serving.

Nutrition Facts

Calories 510, Total Fat 19.6g, Saturated Fat 8.6g, Cholesterol 0mg, Sodium 1322mg, Total Carbohydrate 54.2g, Dietary Fiber 6.6g, Total Sugars 9g, Protein 29.1g

Pumpkin Barley Risotto

Prep time: 10 min Cooking Time: 15 min serve: 2

Ingredients

1 tablespoon butter

1 large onion, finely chopped

½ cup barley

½ teaspoon salt

¼ teaspoon dried parsley

¼ teaspoon black pepper

2 cups vegetable broth

1 cup cubed pumpkin (1/2-inch pieces)

¼ cup grated parmesan cheese plus additional for garnish

Instructions

Press Sauté; heat butter in Instant Pot. Add onion; cook and stir 2 minutes or until softened. Add barley; cook and stir 4 minutes or until barley is translucent. Stir in salt, parsley, and pepper. Add broth and pumpkin; mix well.

Secure lid and move pressure release valve to Sealing. Press Manual or Pressure Cook; cook at High Pressure 6 minutes.

When cooking is complete, press Cancel and use Quick Release.

Press Sauté; adjust heat to low. Cook onion for about 3 minutes or until desired consistency, stirring constantly. Stir in parmesan cheese. Serve immediately with additional cheese.

Nutrition Facts

Calories 320, Total Fat 9.8g, Saturated Fat 5.3g, Cholesterol 20mg, Sodium 1460mg, Total

Carbohydrate 45.9g, Dietary Fiber 9.9g, Total Sugars 5g, Protein 14.3g

Soups and Salads

Easy Keto Tomato Basil Soup

A creamy and delicious low carb tomato soup recipe that takes just minutes to prepare! Keto, Atkins, and gluten free – this is an easy and tasty soup that you can feel great about serving to your family!

Prep Time: 2 minutes Cook Time: 10 minutes Total Time: 12 minutes Servings: 6 servings

Ingredients

1 can (28 ounces) whole plum tomatoes (San Marzano preferred)

2 cups filtered water

1.5 teaspoons coarse kosher salt

1/2 teaspoon onion powder

1/4 teaspoon garlic powder

1 tablespoon butter

8 ounces mascarpone cheese

2 tablespoons granulated erythritol sweetener

1 teaspoon apple cider vinegar

1/4 teaspoon dried basil leaves

1/4 cup prepared basil pesto, plus more for garnish if desired

Instructions

Combine the canned tomatoes, water, salt, onion powder and garlic powder in a medium saucepan.

Bring to a boil over medium-high heat and then simmer for 2 minutes.

Remove from the heat and puree with an immersion blender until smooth (or transfer to a traditional blender and blend, then return blended soup to the pan.)

Return to the stove and add the butter and mascarpone cheese to the soup.

Stir over low heat until melted and creamy – about 2 minutes. Remove from the heat and stir in the sweetener, apple cider vinegar, dried basil, and pesto.

Low Carb Cream of Broccoli & Cheddar Soup

Ingredients

4 cups broccoli florets

2 cups beef broth

1 cup sharp cheddar cheese, shredded

1/2 tsp garlic powder

 1/2 tsp onion powder

1/2 tsp mustard powder

1/8 tsp nutmeg

1/2 tsp kosher salt (or to taste)

1/4 tsp ground black pepper

1/2 cup heavy whipping cream

1/4 cup butter

Instructions

Cook the broccoli florets for 4 minutes in the microwave on high (or steam them on the stove.) Combine the broccoli and other ingredients in a blender and blend until mostly smooth.

Cook on high in the microwave for 2 minutes, stir and cook another 2 minutes, repeat one more time and serve hot.

Alternatively, simmer in a pot on the stove for about 10 minutes. Serve hot.

Nutrition Info

255 calories 22g fat

3g net carbs 7g protein

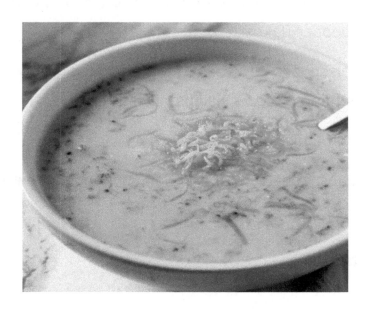

Ginger zucchini noodle egg drop soup

Prep Time: 10 minutes Cook Time: 15 minutes Total Time: 25 minutes Servings: 4-6 servings

Ingredients

4 medium to large zucchini

2 tablespoons extra virgin olive oil 2 tablespoons minced ginger

5 cups shiitake mushrooms, sliced 8 cups vegetable broth, divided

2 cups, plus 1 tablespoon water, divided 1/2 teaspoons red pepper flakes

5 tablespoons low-sodium tamari sauce or soy sauce 2 cups thinly sliced scallions, divided

4 large eggs, beaten

1 tablespoons corn starch Salt & pepper to taste

Instructions

Prepare the zucchini noodles with a spiralizer using the step- by-step guide above.

In a large pot, heat the olive oil over medium-high heat. Add the minced ginger and cook, stirring, for 2 minutes. Add the shiitake mushrooms and a tablespoon of water and cook until the mushrooms begin to sweat. Add 7 cups of the vegetable broth, the remaining water, the red pepper flakes, tamari sauce, and 1½ cups of the chopped scallions. Bring to a boil, stirring occasionally. Meanwhile, mix the remaining cup of vegetable broth with the corn starch and whisk until completely smooth.

While stirring the soup, slowly pour in the beaten eggs in a thin stream. Continue stirring until all of the egg is incorporated. Slowly pour the corn starch mixture into the soup and cook for about 4-5 minutes to thicken. Season to taste with salt & pepper (usually I add just a bit of pepper, but as long, as I'm using a full-sodium vegetable broth, I don't need any extra salt). Add the spiralized zucchini noodles to the pot and cook, stirring, for about 2 minutes, or until the noodles are just soft and flexible (remember, they'll continue cooking in your bowl!). Serve topped with the remaining scallions.

Anti-Inflammatory Egg Drop Soup

Hands-on 10 minutes Total Time: 20 minutes Serving 2 cups/ 480 ml

Ingredients (makes 6 servings)

2 quarts (2 l) chicken stock or vegetable stock or bone broth - you can make your own

1 tbsp freshly grated turmeric or 1 tsp ground turmeric

1 tbsp freshly grated ginger or 1 tsp ground ginger

2 cloves garlic, minced

1 small chile pepper, sliced (14 g/ 0.5 oz) 2 tbsp coconut aminos

2 cups sliced brown mushrooms (144 g/ 5.1 oz)

4 cups chopped Swiss chard or spinach (144 g/ 5.1 oz) 4 large eggs

2 medium spring onions, sliced (30 g/ 1.1 oz) 2 tbsp freshly chopped cilantro

1 tsp salt or to taste (I like pink Himalayan) freshly ground black pepper to taste

6 tbsp extra virgin olive oil (90 ml/ 3 fl oz)

Instructions

Grate the turmeric and ginger root, slice the chile pepper and mince the garlic cloves. Anti-Inflammatory Egg Drop Soup Pour the chicken stock (or vegetable stock) in a large pot and heat over a medium heat, until it starts to simmer. Slice the mushrooms, ... Anti-Inflammatory Egg Drop Soup ... chard stalks and chard leaves. Place the turmeric, ginger, garlic, chile pepper, mushrooms, chard stalks and coconut aminos into the pot and simmer for about 5 minutes. Anti-Inflammatory Egg Drop Soup. Then add the sliced chard leaves and cook for another minute. In a bowl, whisk the eggs and slowly pour them into the simmering soup. Anti-Inflammatory Egg Drop Soup. Keep stirring until the egg is cooked and take off the heat. Chop the cilantro and slice the spring onions. Add them to the pot. Season with salt and pepper to taste. Anti-Inflammatory Egg Drop Soup. Pour into a serving bowl and drizzle with extra virgin olive oil (a tablespoon per serving). Eat immediately or let it cool down and store in an airtight container for up to 5 days.

Soy Bean and Bell Pepper Soup

Ingredients

1 pound dry soy beans

4 cups vegetable stock

1 yellow onion, finely chopped

1 green bell pepper, finely chopped

2 jalapeños, seeds removed and finely chopped

1 cup salsa or diced tomatoes

4 teaspoons minced garlic, about 4 cloves

1 heaping tablespoon chili powder

2 teaspoons ground cumin

2 teaspoons sea salt

1 teaspoon ground pepper

1/2 teaspoon ground cayenne pepper (decrease or omit for a milder soup)

1/2 teaspoon smoked paprika

Avocado and cilantro for topping, if desired

Directions:

Completely submerge the beans in water overnight and make sure there's an inch of water over the beans. Drain the beans and rinse. Put the beans, broth, onion, pepper, jalapeños, salsa, garlic, chili powder, cumin, salt, pepper, cayenne, and paprika in a slow cooker. Stir and combine thoroughly. Cook on high heat for 6 hours until beans are tender. Blend half of the soup until smooth and bring it back to the pot. Top with avocado and cilantro.

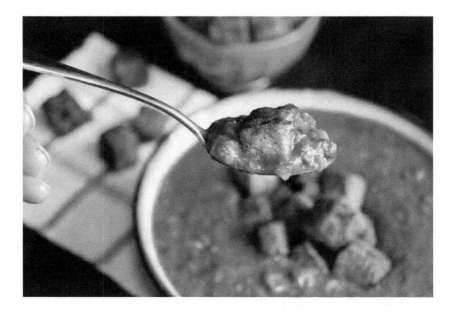

Endive Tomato and Ricotta Cheese Salad

Ingredients:

6 to 7 cups endive,

3 bundles, trimmed

1/4 cucumber, halved lengthwise, then thinly sliced

3 tablespoons chopped or snipped chives

16 cherry tomatoes

1/2 cup sliced almonds

1/4 white onion, sliced

Salt and pepper, to taste

5 ounces ricotta cheese

3 ounces cheddar cheese, shredded

Dressing:

1 sprig cilantro, minced

1 tablespoon distilled white vinegar

1/4 lemon, juiced, about

2 teaspoons

1/4 cup extra-virgin olive oil 1 tsp. egg

free mayonnaise

Directions:

Prep Combine all of the dressing ingredients in a food
processor. Toss with the rest of the ingredients and
combine well.

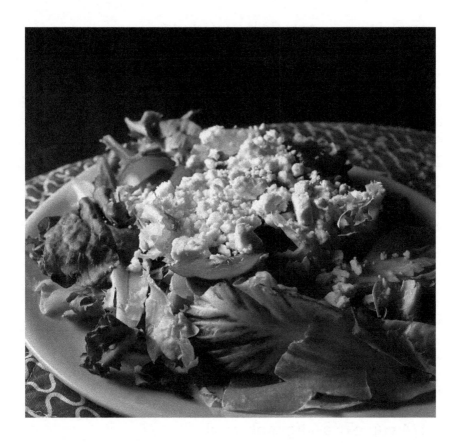

Kale Cucumber Tomatillo and Camambert Salad

Ingredients:

6 to 7 cups kale,

3 bundles, trimmed

1/4 cucumber, halved lengthwise, then thinly sliced

3 tablespoons chopped or snipped chives

16 green tomatillos, sliced in half

1/2 cup sliced almonds

1/4 white onion, sliced

Salt and pepper, to taste

3 ounces cream cheese, crumbled

3 ounces Camembert cheese, crumbled

Dressing 1 sprig of cilantro, minced

1 tablespoon distilled white vinegar

1/4 lemon, juiced, about

2 teaspoons

1/4 cup extra-virgin olive oil

1 tsp. English mustard Prep

Directions:

Combine all of the dressing ingredients in a food processor. Toss with the rest of the ingredients and combine well.

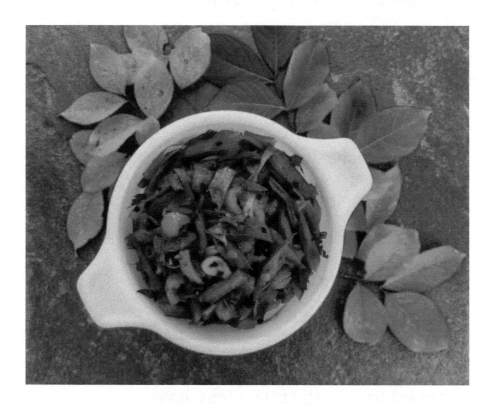

Kale Tomato and Pepperjack Cheese Salad

Ingredients:

6 to 7 cups kale,

3 bundles, trimmed

1/4 cucumber, halved lengthwise, then thinly sliced

3 tablespoons chopped or snipped chives

16 cherry tomatoes

1/2 cup sliced almonds

1/4 white onion, sliced

Salt and pepper, to taste

3 ounces pepper jack cheese, shredded

3 ounces pecorino romano cheese, shredded

Dressing:

1 sprig cilantro, minced

1 tablespoon distilled white vinegar

1/4 lemon, juiced, about 2 teaspoons

1/4 cup extra-virgin olive oil 1 tsp.

Directions:

English mustard Prep Combine all of the dressing ingredients in a food processor. Toss with the rest of the ingredients and combine well.

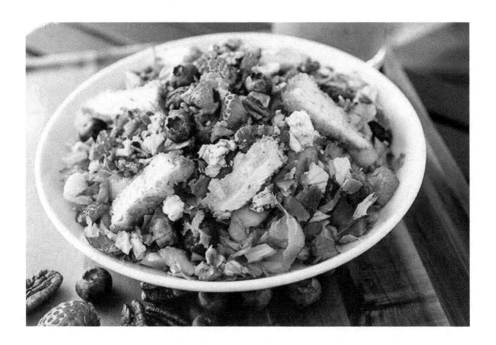

Napa Cabbage Tomatillo and Tofu Ricotta Cheese Salad

Ingredients:

6 to 7 cups napa cabbage,

3 bundles, trimmed

1/4 cucumber, halved lengthwise, then thinly sliced

3 tablespoons chopped or snipped chives

16 green tomatillos, sliced in half

1/2 cup sliced almonds

1/4 white onion, sliced

Salt and pepper, to taste

1 ounce blue cheese, crumbled

6 ounces gouda cheese, shredded

Dressing:

1 sprig cilantro, minced

1 tablespoon distilled white vinegar

1/4 lemon, juiced, about

2 teaspoons

1/4 cup extra-virgin olive oil

1 tsp. egg-free mayonnaise

Directions:

Prep Combine all of the dressing ingredients in a food processor. Toss with the rest of the ingredients and combine well.

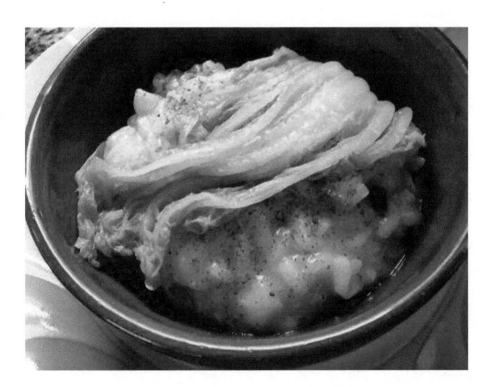

Bib Lettuce Tomatillo and Vegan Parmesan Cheese Salad

Ingredients:

6 to 7 cups bib lettuce,

3 bundles, trimmed

1/4 cucumber, halved lengthwise, then thinly sliced

3 tablespoons chopped or snipped chives

16 tomatillos, sliced in half

1/2 cup sliced almonds

1/4 white onion, sliced

Salt and pepper, to taste

7 ounces parmesan cheese, shredded

1 ounce blue cheese, crumbled

Dressing:

1 sprig cilantro, minced

1 tablespoon distilled white vinegar

1/4 lemon, juiced, about 2 teaspoons

1/4 cup extra-virgin olive oil

Directions:

Prep Combine all of the dressing ingredients in a food processor. Toss with the rest of the ingredients and combine well.

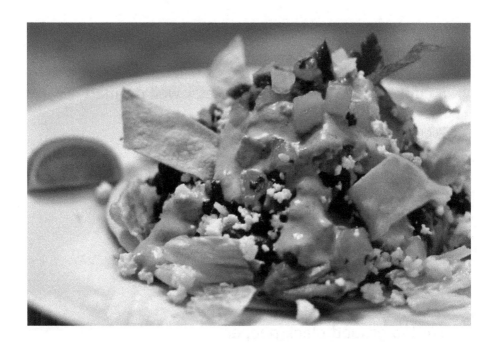

Dinner

Cheesy Cauliflower alla Vodka Casserole

This penne alla vodka recipe uses cauliflower instead of pasta to make it low carb and gluten free. Easy and delicious, it's just as good as the real thing!

Servings: 8 generous 1 cup

Ingredients

8 cups cooked cauliflower florets, well drained

2 cups vodka sauce

2 Tbsp heavy whipping cream

2 Tbsp melted butter

1/3 cup grated Parmesan cheese

1/2 tsp kosher salt

1/4 tsp ground black pepper

6 slices Provolone cheese 1/4 cup fresh basil, chopped

Instructions

Combine the cauliflower, vodka sauce, heavy whipping cream, butter, Parmesan cheese, kosher salt, and black pepper in a large bowl and toss to coat well.

Transfer into a 9 x 13 baking dish (or equivalent) and top with slices of Provolone (or mozzarella) cheese.

Bake in a preheated 375 degree (F) oven for 30 – 40 minutes or until the casserole is bubbling and the cheese is completely melted.

Remove from the oven and let it rest for about 10 minutes. Top with chopped fresh basil and serve.

Nutrition Info

214 calories, 14g fat, 6g net carbs, 12g protein

Caprese Style Portobellos

Servings: 4

Ingredients

Large portobello mushroom caps, gills removed

Cherry tomatoes, halved

Shredded or fresh mozzarella (although I've tried both I prefer the dryer shredded version for this because of the moisture factor seeping out)

Fresh basil

Olive oil

Instructions

Heat oven to 400 degrees.

Line a baking sheet with foil for easy clean up.

Brush the caps and rims with olive oil on each mushroom.

Slice cherry or grape tomatoes in half, place in a bowl, drizzle with olive oil, add chopped basil, salt and pepper. Let it sit for a few minutes to let the flavors meld. Place your cheese on the bottom of the mushroom cap, spoon on the tomato basil mixture and bake until cheese melts and mushrooms are cooked but not overcooked.

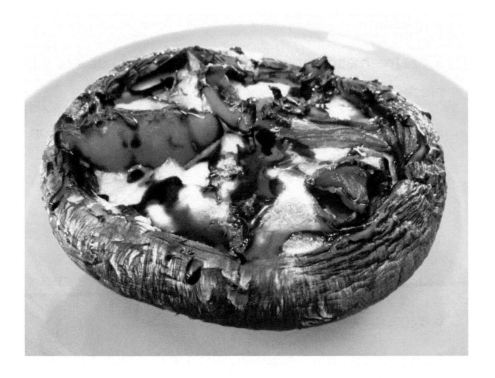

Asparagus and Tomato Frittata with Havarti and Dill

When asparagus goes on sale in the spring, This Asparagus and Tomato Frittata with Havarti and Dill is a perfect thing to make for breakfast, lunch, or dinner!

Prep Time 10 minutes Cook Time 20 minutes Total Time 30 minutes Servings 6 servings

Ingredients

8 oz. fresh asparagus, ends trimmed and cut into small pieces

2 tsp. olive oil (or maybe a little more, depending on your pan)

2/3 cup diced cherry tomatoes

1 tsp. dried dill weed (see notes)

4 oz. Havarti cheese, cut into small cubes (see notes)

6 eggs, beaten well

Spike seasoning, Vege-Sal, and fresh ground black pepper to taste for seasoning eggs (see notes)

sliced green onions for garnish (optional, but good)

Instructions

Cut off the woody ends of the asparagus spears, then cut asparagus into pieces about 1 1/2 inches long.

Heat oil in heavy frying pan over medium-high heat, add asparagus and cook 3-4 minutes.

While asparagus cooks, dice the cherry tomatoes into halves (or fourths if they're large) and dice the cheese into small pieces.

After asparagus has cooked for 3-4 minutes, add the cherry tomatoes and dill weed (affiliate link) and cook for 1-2 minutes more.

Break eggs into a bowl and beat well.

When tomatoes have cooked for 2 minutes, pour eggs over, season with Spike Seasoning (affiliate link) and Vege-Sal (affiliate link) or salt, and fresh ground black pepper.

Then sprinkle cheese over the top. (There will be some pieces of asparagus and tomatoes poking up at this point, but the frittata will puff up more as it cooks.)

Start to preheat the broiler

Cover pan and cook on low heat about 8-10 minutes, or until eggs are set and the cheese is completely melted on the top.

Put frittata under the broiler for a few minutes, checking carefully to see when it's starting to get brown.

When the top is browned to your liking, cut frittata into six wedges, garnish with sliced green onions, and serve hot.

Nutrition Info

Calories: 180 Total Fat: 13g Saturated Fat: 6g

Unsaturated Fat: 6g Cholesterol: 235mg Sodium: 322mg Carbohydrates: 4g

Cheesy Vegetarian Spaghetti Squash Lasagna

Prep Time 10 minutes Cook Time 1 hour

Total Time 1 hour 10 minutes

Servings 2 servings

Ingredients

1 large spaghetti squash (approx. 3 lbs) olive oil for drizzling

1/2 cup onion (white or yellow)

1-2 cloves garlic, smashed and minced

5 oz mushrooms (approx. 2 cups chopped)

2-3 oz fresh spinach (approx. 1.5 cups chopped) 1 plum tomato, chopped

1.5 cups ricotta cheese 1 egg white

1/3-1/2 cup freshly grated parmesan cheese to taste

1 tsp Italian seasoning blend (I love using Mrs. Dash) 1/2 tsp dried basil

1/2 tsp garlic powder salt and pepper to taste 1/2 cup spaghetti sauce 2 oz grated mozzarella

crushed red pepper flakes to taste

Instructions

Pre-heat oven to 400 degrees F.

Slice your spaghetti squash in half lengthwise and scoop out the seeds.

For easy cutting, feel free to microwave for 4-5 minutes to soften it up just a tad. The knife slides through much easier this way!

Next grab a lipped baking sheet or a rimmed baking dish. Rub the cut side of the squash with a teeny bit of olive oil.

Place inside a baking dish or atop rimmed baking sheet and roast face-down for about 40 minutes, or until tender and easily pierced with a fork.

Cooking time will vary a bit depending on the size of your squash so adjust accordingly. Once ready, the once rock-hard exterior of the squash will be visibly softened with a tender interior.

While the squash roasts, start prepping your cheese and veggies.

Chop your onion, garlic, mushrooms, spinach and tomato, separately, then set aside.

Bring a pan or skillet to medium-high heat with a drizzle of olive oil.

Sauté onion until tender and slightly golden, then add garlic and mushrooms and continue to cook until softened. Set aside. In a large bowl, combine ricotta, egg white, freshly grated parmesan cheese, fresh chopped spinach, Italian seasoning, basil, and garlic powder.

Drain your mushroom/onion mixture and add to the bowl along with your chopped tomato.

Mix well, adding a little salt and pepper to taste.

Once your squash is ready, allow to cool slightly, then use a fork to separate the squash's interior into spaghetti-like strands. Remove, a little of the squash, will help you better stuff these bad boys.

Take a little out and add your filling to the squash, swirling to mix.

Top with remaining spaghetti squash strands and stir.

Next add a few spoonfuls of your favorite spaghetti sauce on top and finish off with your grated mozzarella cheese. Add extra of either if desired.

Add an optional pinch of crushed red pepper flakes on top (skip if sensitive to heat) and bake at 350 degrees F for around 20 minutes until hot and bubbly.

For golden flecks of mozzarella, switch oven to broil on HIGH for 2 minutes at the end and remove once bubbling.

Serve piping hot with a healthy side salad or roasted veggies for a balanced meal that's sure to rock your plate! Enjoy!

Recipe Notes

For a casserole style lasagna, spritz a baking dish with olive oil and add your forked strands of spaghetti squash, top with cheese and veggie filling and mix. Add a layer of red sauce and cheese (as much or as little as your heart desires of each) and bake at 350 F until hot and bubbly, approx. 20-25 minutes.

Depending on sizing and availability, you can use two smaller spaghetti squash in place of one large squash.

Nutrition Info

Calories 695

Calories from Fat 342 Fat 38g

Saturated Fat 22g Cholesterol 128mg Sodium 1055mg Potassium 1479mg Carbohydrates 54g Fiber 11g

Sugar 21g Protein 43g

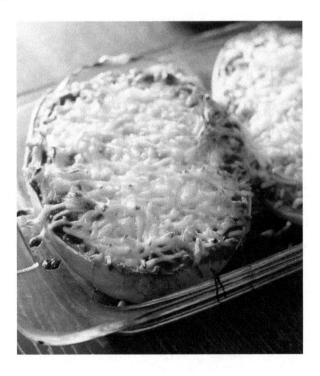

Red Rice with Vegan Chorizo and Tomatoes

Ingredients

1 poblano chili, diced

1 red onion, diced

1/2 cup vegan Chorizo (Soyrizo), crumbled

1 ½ cups garbanzo beans, drained

1 cup uncooked red rice

1 ½ cups chopped tomatoes

½ cup water

4 tbsp. chimichurri sauce

1/2 tsp. cayenne pepper

Sea salt Black pepper

Toppings: fresh coriander (cilantro), chopped spring onions, sliced avocado, guacamole, etc.

Directions:

Combine all the burrito bowl ingredients (not toppings) in a slow cooker. Cook on low for 3 hours, or until the rice is cooked. Serve hot with topping ingredients

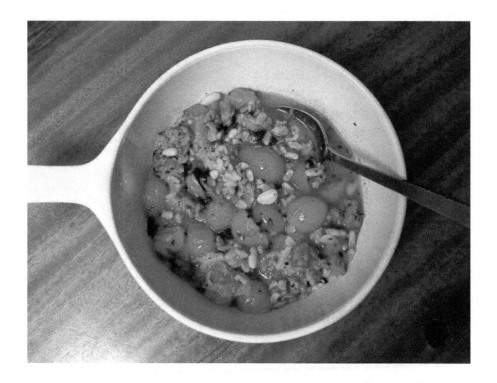

White Bean & Vegan Chorizo Burrito

Ingredients

1 ancho chili, diced

1 red onion, diced

1 mild red chili, finely chopped

1 1/2 cup white beans

1 cup uncooked white rice

1 1/2 cups chopped tomatoes

1/2 cup water

1/4 cup vegan chorizos, coarsely chopped

1/2 cup meatless meatballs, crumbled

1 tsp. dried thyme

Sea salt Black pepper

Toppings: fresh coriander (cilantro), chopped spring onions, sliced avocado, guacamole, etc.

Directions:

Combine all the burrito bowl ingredients (not toppings) in a slow cooker. Cook on low for 3 hours, or until the rice is cooked. Serve hot with topping ingredients

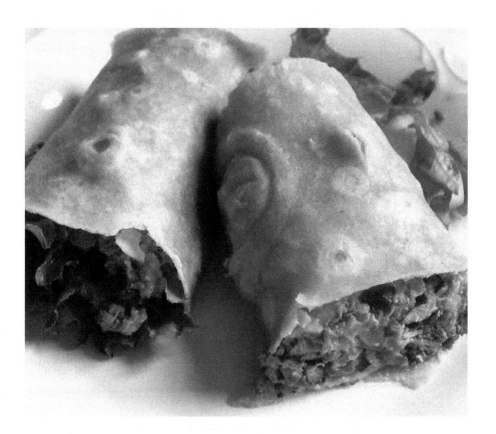

Parmesan Cauliflower Steak

Servings: 4 Servings

Ingredients

1 large head cauliflower 4 tbsp butter

2 tbsp Urban Accents Manchego and Roasted Garlic seasoning blend

1/4 cup parmesan cheese Salt and pepper to taste

Instructions

Preheat oven to 400 degrees Remove leaves from cauliflower Slice cauliflower lengthwise through core into 1 inch steaks (mine made about 4) Melt butter in microwave and mix with seasoning blend to make paste

Brush mixture over steaks and season with salt and pepper to taste Heat non-stick pan over medium and place cauliflower steaks for 2-3 minutes until lightly browned Flip carefully, repeat. Place cauliflower steaks on lined baking sheet. Bake cauliflower steaks in oven for 15-20 minutes until golden and tender. Sprinkle with parmesan cheese and serve.

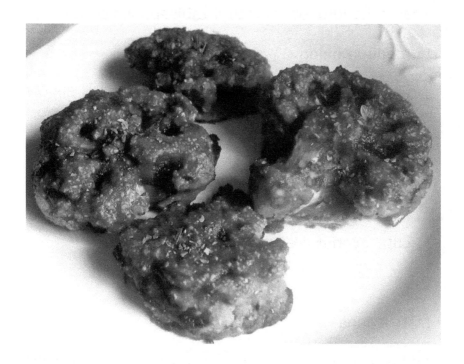

Vegetarian Red Coconut Curry

Servingss 2 servings

Ingredients

1 cup broccoli florets

1 large handful of spinach 4 tablespoons coconut oil

¼ medium onion

1 teaspoon minced garlic 1 teaspoon minced ginger 2 teaspoons Fysh sauce

2 teaspoons soy sauce

1 tablespoon red curry paste

½ cup coconut cream (or coconut milk)

Instructions

Add 2 tbsp. coconut oil to a pan and bring to medium-high heat.

Chop onions and mince garlic while you wait. When the oil is hot, add the onion to the pan and let it sizzle.

Allow it to cook for 3-4 minutes to caramelize and become semi-translucent. Once this happens, add the garlic to the pan and let it brown slightly. About 30 seconds.

Turn the heat to medium-low and add broccoli florets to the pan. aStir everything together well. Let the broccoli take on the flavors of the onion and garlic. This should take about 1-2 minutes. Move everything in your pan to the side and add 1 tbsp. red curry paste. You want this hitting the bottom of the pan so that all of the flavors can be released from the spices. Once your red curry paste starts to smell pungent, mix everything together again and add a large handful of spinach over the top. Once the spinach begins to wilt, add coconut cream and mix together. Stir everything together and then add 2 tbsp. more coconut oil, 2 tsp. fysh sauce, 2 tsp. soy sauce, and 1 tsp. minced ginger. Let this simmer for 5-10 minutes, depending on how thick you want the sauce. Dish out and serve! Feel free to garnish with a few slices of red cabbage and black sesame seeds for color.

Nutrition Info

398 Calories 40.73g Fats 7.86g Carbs

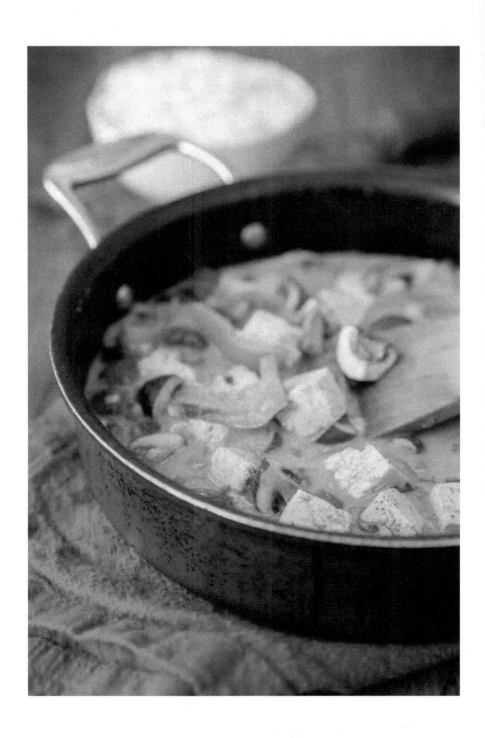

Sweets

Apple Pie Quinoa Pudding

Prep time: 5 min Cooking Time: 10 min serve: 2

Ingredients

2 cups quinoa

2 cups apples finely chopped

1 cup soy milk

½ tablespoon cinnamon powder

½ tablespoon Vanilla free

1/8 teaspoon ground cardamom

½ cup golden dates

Instructions

Place all Ingredients in the Instant Pot.

Cook on manual at high pressure for 10 minutes. When time is up, quickly release the pressure.

Serve and enjoy! This is delicious served hot, warm or cold.

Nutrition Facts

Calories 251, Total Fat 2.7g, Saturated Fat 0.3g, Cholesterol 0mg , Sodium 34mg, Total Carbohydrate 50.5g, Dietary Fiber 6.8g, Total Sugars 28.4g, Protein 5.9g

Baked Peaches

Prep time: 10 min Cooking Time: 15 min serve: 2

Ingredients

1/8 cup apricots

1/8 cup dates chopped

1/8 cup walnuts chopped

1 teaspoon nutmeg

1 tablespoon honey

4 small peaches

2 tablespoons coconut oil

1 cup Water

Instructions

In a small bowl, mix apricots, dates, walnuts, nutmeg and honey.

Using a paring knife, remove the peaches cores, leaving the bottom 1/2 inch of the peaches.

Fill apples with filling mixture and top each with a thin slice of butter.

Pour 2/3 cup water in the Instant Pot and arrange the apples in the bottom of the pot. Add any extra butter to the cooking water.

Secure the lid, making sure the vent is closed.

Use the display panel to select the Manual or Pressure Cook function. Use the + /- keys and program the Instant Pot for 3 minutes.

When the time is up, let the pressure naturally release for 5 minutes, quickly releasing the remaining pressure.

Serve warm.

Nutrition Facts

Calories 299, Total Fat 14.9g, Saturated Fat 12.1g, Cholesterol 0mg, Sodium 4mg, Total Carbohydrate

38.3g, Dietary Fiber 5g , Total Sugars 37.8g, Protein 3g

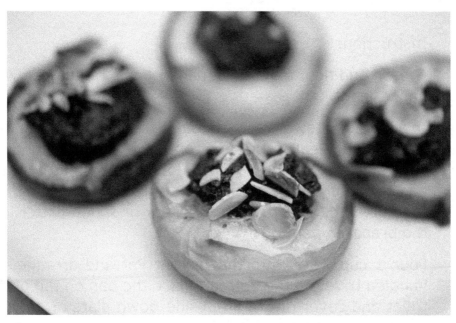

Simple White Cake

Prep time: 10 min Cooking Time: 30 min serve: 2
Ingredients

1 tablespoon coconut sugar

½ tablespoon coconut oil

1 egg

1/8 teaspoon vanilla extract

½ cup coconut flour

½ teaspoon baking powder

1/8 cup coconut milk

Instructions

Grease and flour a 9x9-inch pan or line a muffin pan with paper liners.

In a medium bowl, cream together the coconut sugar and coconut oil. Beat in the egg, one at a time, then stir in the vanilla. Combine coconut flour and baking powder, add to the creamed mixture and mix well. Finally stir in the milk until batter is smooth. Pour or spoon batter into the prepared pan.

Pour 1 cup water into the Instant Pot and arrange the handled trivet on the bottom. Place the pan on top of the trivet and cover it with an upside-down plate or another piece of parchment to protect the brownies from condensation.

Secure the lid and move the steam release valve to Sealing. Select Manual/Pressure Cook to cook on high pressure for 30 minutes. When the cooking cycle is complete, let the pressure naturally release for 10 minutes, then move the steam release valve to Venting to release any remaining pressure. When the floating valve drops, remove the lid.

Let cool slightly before serving

Nutrition Facts

Calories 260, Total Fat 12.2g,Saturated Fat 8.8g, Cholesterol 82mg, Sodium 54mg, Total Carbohydrate 31.1g, Dietary Fiber 12.4g , Total Sugars 0.7g, Protein 7.6g

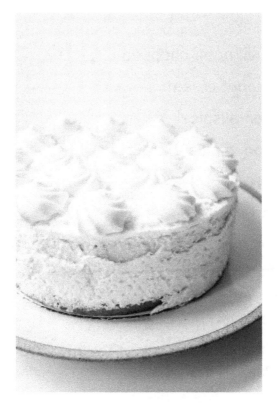

Brazil nuts Cake

Prep time: 05 min Cooking Time: 40 min serve: 2

Ingredients

1-1/2 tablespoons sugar-free chocolate chips

2 tablespoons butter melted

1 egg

1 cup all-purpose flour

½ tablespoon arrowroot powder

½ teaspoon baking powder

½ teaspoon pumpkin purée organic

¼ cup honey

¼ cup Brazil nuts, chopped

¼ cup coconut cream

½ teaspoon allspice

¼ teaspoon vanilla extract

Instruction

In a large bowl, thoroughly mix all ingredients, until a perfectly even mixture is obtained.

Next, pour 1 cup filtered water into the Instant Pot and insert the trivet.

Transfer the mixture from the bowl into a well-greased, Instant Pot– friendly pan.

Using a sling if desired, place the pan onto the trivet, and cover loosely with aluminium foil. Close the lid, set the pressure release to Sealing, and select Manual/Pressure Cook. Set the Instant Pot to 40 minutes on high pressure, and

Once cooked, let the pressure naturally disperse from the Instant Pot for about 10 minutes, then carefully switch the pressure release to Venting.

Open the Instant Pot and remove the pan. Allow to cool completely before serving. Serve, and enjoy!

Nutrition Facts

Calories 470, Total Fat 10g, Saturated Fat 7.1g, Cholesterol 82mg, Sodium 40mg, Total Carbohydrate

85.5g, Dietary Fiber 2.6g, Total Sugars 36.2g, Protein 10.1g

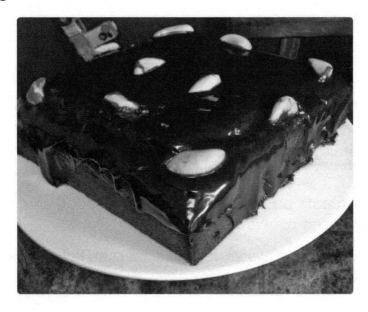

Oatmeal Raisin Cookies

Prep time: 15 min Cooking Time: 20 min serve: 2

Ingredients

1 tablespoon coconut oil

1 tablespoon honey

1 egg

1/8 teaspoon vanilla extract

1cup coconut flour

1/8 teaspoon baking soda

1/8 teaspoon ground nutmeg

1/8 teaspoon salt

1 cup rolled oats

1 tablespoon raisins

Instructions

In large bowl, cream together coconut oil, honey, until smooth.

Beat in the egg and vanilla until fluffy. Stir together coconut flour, baking soda, nutmeg, and salt. Gradually beat into butter mixture.

Stir in oats and raisins. Drop by teaspoon complete onto ungreased cookie sheets.

1 cup filtered water into the Instant Pot and insert the trivet.

Transfer the mixture from the bowl into a well-greased, Instant Pot– friendly pan.

Using a sling if desired, place the pan onto the trivet, Close the lid, set the pressure release to Sealing, and select Manual/Pressure Cook. Set the Instant Pot to 20 minutes on High pressure, and

Once cooked, let the pressure naturally disperse from the Instant Pot for about 10 minutes, then carefully switch the pressure release to Venting.

Nutrition Facts

Calories 273, Total Fat 8.9g, Saturated Fat 5.5g, Cholesterol 41mg, Sodium 129mg, Total Carbohydrate

40.1g, Dietary Fiber 14.2g , Total Sugars 6g, Protein 8.2g

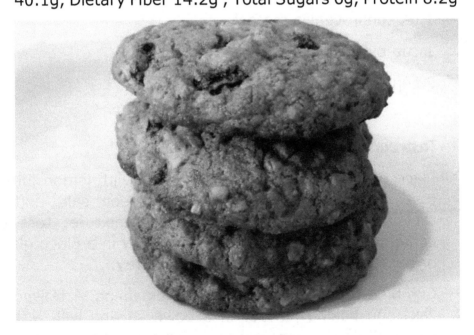

Blueberry-Peach Cobbler

(Prep time: 20 min| Cooking Time: 60 min | serve: 2)

Ingredients

5 peaches, peeled, pitted, and sliced

2 tablespoons fresh lemon juice

1 cup coconut sugar, divided

Pinch salt,

2 cups coconut flour, divided

1 teaspoon baking powder

½ cup coconut oil,

2 large eggs

1 teaspoon vanilla extract

1 cup buttermilk

2 cups fresh blueberries

Instructions

Place peaches in a large bowl. Drizzle with lemon juice; toss. Add coconut sugar, 1/8 teaspoon salt, and 2 tablespoons coconut flour to peach mixture; toss to combine. Arrange peach mixture evenly in a 8inch glass or baking dish coated with cooking spray.

Combine reaming coconut flour, remaining ¼ teaspoon salt, and baking powder in a bowl, stirring well with a whisk. Place the remaining coconut sugar and coconut oil in a medium bowl, and beat with a mixer at medium speed until light and fluffy (about 2 minutes). Add egg, 1 at a time, beating well after each addition. Stir in vanilla extract. Add flour mixture and buttermilk, beating just until combined. Stir in blueberries.

Spread batter evenly over peach mixture;

Pour 1 cup filtered water into the Instant Pot and insert the trivet.

Using a sling if desired, place the pan onto the trivet, Close the lid, set the pressure release to sealing, and select Manual/Pressure Cook. Set the Instant Pot to 55 minutes on High pressure, and Once cooked, let the pressure naturally disperse from the Instant Pot for about 10 minutes, then carefully switch the pressure release to Venting.

Nutrition Facts

Calories 346, Total Fat 18.6g, Saturated Fat 14.4g, Cholesterol 48mg , Sodium 76mg, Total Carbohydrate 38.4g, Dietary Fiber 14.4g , Total Sugars 14.1g, Protein 7.9g

Coconut-Blackberries Flaxseed Pudding

Prep time: 10 min Cooking Time: 05 min serve: 2

Ingredients

½ cup almond milk

½ cup Water

½ cup blackberries

½ cup flex seeds

½ cup quinoa

1/8 cup honey

¼ teaspoon pure vanilla extract

Fresh berries for garnish

Instructions

Combine the almond milk, water, blackberries, flex seeds, quinoa, honey, and vanilla extract in the inner pot.

Lock the lid into place. Select Pressure Cook or Manual; set the pressure to High and the time to 3 minutes. Make sure the steam release knob is in the sealed position. After cooking, naturally release the pressure for 5 minutes, then quick release any remaining pressure.

Unlock and remove the lid. Pour the pudding into individual serving cups and refrigerate until it sets, about 1 hour.

Serve cold garnished with blackberries.

Baked Quinoa

Prep time: 10 min Cooking Time: 70 min serve: 2

Ingredients

½ tablespoon avocado oil

½ tablespoon honey

1egg

1 tablespoon almond butter

¼ cup coconut milk

¼ teaspoon Vanilla

½ cup Quinoa

¼ teaspoon baking powder

Pinch salt

1/8 cup chocolate chips

Powdered sugar for garnish

Instructions

In a medium bowl, beat together avocado oil and honey. Add egg a time and beat until uniform.

Add almond butter, coconut milk and vanilla and stir to combine.

In a large bowl, stir together quinoa, baking powder and salt. Add wet Ingredients and mix until fully incorporated.

Fold in chocolate chips.

Coat the inside of a 7-inch baking pan or casserole with non-stick spray-

Spread batter in pan and cover pan with foil.

Pour one cup of water in the Instant Pot and insert the steam rack. Lower the pan or casserole on to the steam rack, secure the lid, and make sure the vent is closed.

Use the display panel to select the Manual or Pressure Cook function. Use the + /- keys and program the Instant Pot for 45 minutes.

When the time is up, let the pressure naturally release for 15 minutes, quickly releasing the remaining pressure.

Carefully remove the pan and allow to cool for 10 minutes before serving.

Garnish with powdered sugar (optional). Keep covered and serve

Nutrition Facts

Calories 392, Total Fat 20g, Saturated Fat 9.9g, Cholesterol 84mg , Sodium 125mg, Total Carbohydrate

41.7g, Dietary Fiber 5g, Total Sugars 11.3g, Protein 12g

Rich Antioxidant Cheesecake

Prep time:15 min Cooking Time: 25 min serve: 2

Ingredients

Base

½ cup feta cheese softened

1-1/2 teaspoon coconut flour

1-1/2 tablespoons coconut cream

1 egg

½ tablespoon moringa powder

¼ teaspoon vanilla extract

Topping

1/8 cup brown sugar

1/2 cup coconut cream

Instructions

Combine the feta cheese, coconut flour, coconut cream, egg, moringa powder, and vanilla in a large bowl. Mix thoroughly. Place mixture in spring form pan, then loosely cover with aluminium foil. 2. Pour 2 cups filtered water into Instant Pot, then add trivet, placing the spring form pan atop the rack.

Move the valve to Sealing and close the lid of the Instant Pot.

Set to Manual/Pressure Cook, and let cook for 25 minutes at High pressure. Once cooked, let the pressure naturally disperse from the Instant Pot for about 10 minutes, then carefully switch the pressure release to Venting.

Remove pan, and let cool for 30 minutes. Then refrigerate for at least 45 minutes (a few hours is preferable).

Remove foil. Mix the brown sugar and coconut cream in a small bowl, spread evenly on the cake before serving. Store any remaining cheesecake in the refrigerator.

Nutrition Facts

Calories 192, Total Fat 12.1g, Saturated Fat 8g, Cholesterol 115mg, Sodium 456mg, Total Carbohydrate 13.2g, Dietary Fiber 0.9g , Total Sugars 10.8g, Protein 8.7g

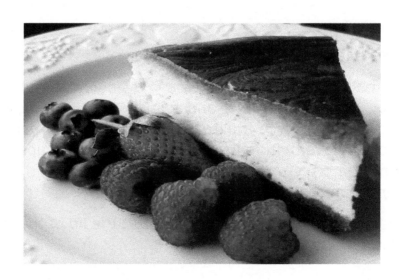

Lemon curd & blueberry loaf cake

Prep: 20 mins Cook:1 hr and 15 mins easy Cuts into 8-10 slices

Ingredients

175g softened butter

500ml tub Greek yogurt (you need 100ml/3.5fl oz in the cake, the rest to serve)

300g jar good lemon curd (you need 2 tbsp in the cake, the rest to serve)

3 eggs zest and juice 1 lemon, plus extra zest to serve

200g self-raising flour 175g golden caster sugar

200g punnet of blueberries (you need 85g/3oz in the cake, the rest to serve) 140g icing sugar

edible flowers, such as purple or yellow primroses, to serve (optional)

Directions:

1 Heat oven to 160C/140C fan/gas 3. Grease a 2lb loaf tin and line with a long strip of baking parchment. Put 100g yogurt, 2 tbsp lemon curd, the softened butter, eggs, lemon zest, flour and caster sugar into a large mixing bowl. Quickly mix with an electric whisk until the batter just comes together. Scrape half into the prepared tin. Weigh 85g blueberries from the punnet and sprinkle half into the tin, scrape the rest of the batter on top, then scatter the other half of the 85g berries. Bake for 1 hr 10 mins-1 hr 15 mins until golden, and a skewer poked into the centre comes out clean. 2 Cool in the tin, then

carefully lift onto a serving plate to ice. Sift the icing sugar into a bowl and stir in enough lemon juice to make a thick, smooth icing. Spread over the top of the cake, then decorate with lemon zest and edible flowers, if you like. Serve in slices with extra lemon curd, Greek yogurt and blueberries.

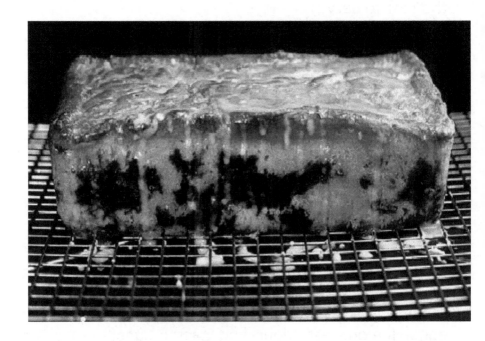

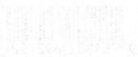